TERRY MARCHANT

How to Survive a Gym Membership

With thirty-five years of experience, I have witnessed people's failures with their exercise programs in gyms, and I have some answers.

First edition

This book was professionally typeset on Reedsy.
Find out more at reedsy.com

I never met a gym I didnt like!

Contents

1

Introduction

I was first exposed to exercise when I graduated from high school in the 70s. I wasn't involved in sports while in school, so it was a new experience for me. One week, I was in high school, and a week later, I was working in a local factory. From there, I met a couple of brothers, and they would get together several times a week and lift weights. That's what they called it back then. We didn't have gyms you could join.

We met at a local church that had weights in the basement. Barbells, dumbbells, curl bars etc. They invited me to join them and I really took to it. We were consistent, and I actually put on a few pounds of muscle. It was a great experience because these guys had been doing it for years and I got to learn from them. After that, it was up to finding a garage with a bench press and a curl bar. It was always fun to me and I liked being healthy.

Gyms started popping up in the late eighties to early ninties and I joined one in a nearby town. I would get there in the evenings to lift weights, and the weight room would be busy, so I couldn't get in. But they had these exercise machines, which I would later get to know as Nautilus Stations. Not many people were using them, so they were open to use. This would turn out to be a huge advantage. From this, I learned to use the Nautilus-type machines instead of the free weights most people believe you have to use.

Since those times, I have had gym memberships for most of my adult life. So, I have observed how new people in a gym fail, and over time have formed some thoughts on how people can put the odds of success in their favor. The success rate for new members has to be pretty low. I would see new people come in all excited about exercising, and then in a few weeks, you wouldn't see them anymore. I was lucky in that I had seen from an early age some success and, from that, developed some good habits. And then I kept repeating them.

I have been doing the same type of workout all these years. People claim you have to mix things up. I am sure that is true for an athlete. But if you are a busy person trying to stay healthy, stick with something that works. I can assure you that if you do this consistently, it will produce muscle tone, and you will be healthy.

I want to clarify who I am writing this for. Mainly people over thirty-five but really anyone unable to keep a program for any length of time. Most people will get a membership, last two, four, or six weeks, and give up for whatever reason. And then there are the pretty serious, knowledgeable people who can last three months or so and then stop and not come back or at least not come back for some time. Starts and stops are part of the deal when you look at it over a lifetime. I think of it in percentages' and that is my goal, to give you the information you need to put the odds in your favor. This is not for young athletes, serious weight lifters, or bodybuilders. However, at some point, everyone will come to a point where they will need this type of program. Take serious athletes who believe all workouts must last two to three hours. When they get to a point where they can no longer do this, they quit completely instead of adjusting to something doable.

2

Why Exercise

In my younger days, I lifted weights to gain muscle, mainly because I had a slim build. I could never get past that in those days, but at least I could get some muscle tone. I was able to put on a few pounds. Of course, age brought some weight, and without exercise, I could have accepted poor health like everyone else. Along with everything that comes with it, like back issues, being overweight, and all that unpleasant stuff I never got to experience!

As I got older, I switched from using free weights for muscle to using Nautilus Stations for health. This took place when gyms became available in the eighties. My workouts became shorter in time as I focused on half a dozen stations. Anyway, I think it's important for you to understand your chances of having a successful workout program increase dramatically when your focus or reason for exercising changes from building muscle or losing/gaining weight to simply getting healthy. Then you allow time in the gym to achieve the goals you have.

This is where I want to define what I consider a successful

workout program to be. That is a program you can do week after week, month after month, year after year, and decade after decade. Never go over three weeks without getting to the gym. For me, it is more like two weeks. Because it just doesn't happen. I always had a clock in my head that said, "Hey, it's time to get to the gym". So, time in the gym will allow you to accomplish what you seek, such as muscle tone or weight loss. One huge advantage to me was that I had a bad knee from an early age from a basketball injury. As long as I exercised, it didn't bother me. If I went two to three weeks without exercising, it would let me know it was time to get in there. The muscles and tendons in my knee benefited from the exercise.

Another huge driver for me was simply feeling younger. When I was forty, I loved the fact that I felt like a twenty-five-year-old. When I was fifty, I felt like a thirty-five-year-old. When I was 60, I felt like a forty-five-year-old. How much value can you put on something like that? This is huge!

Do you want another reason for having a successful exercise program? How about avoiding the doctor or hospitals? Both my parents had heart disease and diabetes, so you can't always avoid them completely, but life choices can definitely make a difference. I am currently in my late sixties, and I have been admitted to a hospital once for a colonoscopy. I consider that to be a pretty good record.

Another reason for exercising is it reduces stress. To me, that is just a part of feeling healthy. Being able to sleep well. Being able to move a couch without tearing a muscle. Being able to walk up a set of stairs without getting winded. I was pre-diabetic for what seemed like twenty years. Because of my exercise program and eating habits, I was able to put diabetes off for that long, and then once I was considered a diabetic, it was easily handled.

This is major stuff here!

3

Gym or Home Equipment

I am sure there are some people who can have a successful exercise program from home equipment, but month after month, year after year, decade after decade, and never going over two to three weeks without exercising? The issue with exercising from home is the fact that it is so easy to be distracted. You are much more likely to be interrupted at home than at a gym. And it is much easier to just blow it off from home. All home equipment becomes a coat rack eventually.

For me the biggest factor was if I paid for the monthly fee at a gym, I would be much more likely to attend it. And remember, the key to success is putting the odds in your favor.

You also have to consider how well a modern gym is equipped. Not many homes would be able to match what a well-equipped gym can offer in the way of options for use.

Choosing between gym and home equipment depends on your personal preferences, goals, and lifestyle. Here are some key points to consider for each option:

Gym Equipment

Pros:

- **Variety:** Gyms offer a wide range of equipment, from cardio machines to free weights and specialized machines.
- **Social Environment:** Working out in a gym can be motivating due to the presence of other fitness enthusiasts.
- **Professional Guidance:** Access to personal trainers and fitness classes can help you stay on track and learn proper techniques.

Cons:

- **Cost:** Gym memberships can be expensive, especially if you don't use the facilities regularly.
- **Travel Time:** Commuting to and from the gym can be time-consuming.
- **Crowds:** Gyms can be crowded, especially during peak hours, which might limit your access to equipment.

Home Equipment
Pros:

- **Convenience:** You can work out anytime without leaving your home, making it easier to fit exercise into your schedule.
- **Cost-Effective:** While the initial investment might be high, it can save money in the long run compared to gym memberships.
- **Privacy:** You can exercise in a private setting without feeling self-conscious.

Cons:

- **Limited Equipment:** Home gyms might not have the same variety of equipment as commercial gyms.
- **Space:** Setting up a home gym requires space, which might be a constraint for some people.

Best of Both Worlds

Some people prefer a hybrid approach, using both gym and home equipment to maximize their workout options. For example, you might use the gym for specialized equipment and social interaction while using home equipment for convenience and flexibility. I personally use the hybrid approach, doing stretching exercises at home. The older you get, the more important stretching becomes.

4

Membership Killers

Like I said I have had gym memberships most of my adult life. This time was mostly spent in three separate gyms, and I have fond memories of each one of them. This is a span of around thirty-five years. I once said, "I never met a gym I didn't like". Why not? All three were well equipped with plenty of room and quality workstations to handle the number of participants. So, in all that time, I observed new people coming in full of excitement and anticipation of bettering their lives, only to succumb to leaving in a few weeks or months. In my mind, that is or can be part of the process. A workout program is built around starts and stops.

It's not like I was in a gym continually throughout those years. There were times when things would come up, and I would miss it for a month or two, and then I would be right back in there where I left off. And there were a couple of key points that allowed me to do that. Number one was the fact that I was doing it for one thing! Health! And it always paid off in big ways. Well worth the cost and the effort. I always maintained a healthy weight. Was never harnessed with the normal health issues most people encounter. I was able to accomplish that because I wasn't doing it to build muscle or to participate in weightlifting tournaments. When you bring those kinds of things into the equation, you drop your chance of succeeding tremendously!!

I have been fortunate in that I had easy access to a gym. The first gym I had was a 20-minute drive to get to. For twenty-some years, I had a membership in the town where I worked. It was almost thirty minutes from my house, but I could go to the gym after work. Now I am fortunate to have one a few blocks away. You will have to decide how far you will go to accomplish your goals. I am going to give you a blueprint that will increase your odds of succeeding. But for now, I will lay out a few membership killers that stop new people in their tracks when entering a gym for the first time, the second time, or the third time, etc.

I am killing it at the gym: A lot of people come into a gym with heightened expectations of getting into great shape in a short time period. That is possible, but I ask you, what are the percentages? If you have never exercised regularly, it is not going to happen. These are the people who will do twenty to thirty different exercises or "sets" and spend one to three hours at a workout. This is not for the inexperienced! The issue is you will run out of energy in a short period of time. Or the long workouts will eventually cause you to stop because how long can you take two to three hours a day out of your schedule? There are three main ingredients to a successful exercise program. I will go into these in-depth later on, but for now, here is the list: Time, energy, and a good plan. How long can a normal person spend two to three hours at a gym? To do this you would have to sleep twelve hours and spend the rest of the day eating to come up with enough energy to carry this out. Of course, that is a bit of an exaggeration but I hope you get my point. Workouts should be short, thirty-five minutes to an hour max, and use five to six different stations. Allowing a period of committed time there to bring the results you are looking for as opposed to doing it in a short period of time. My workouts last thirty-five minutes.

Gang memberships: What I am referring to is the practice of joining a gym with other people. Some will get together as two or three people or more to exercise together. This sounds good but is very hard to pull off! There will always be things that come up to cause one or more of your group to miss, and then you won't go because of it. Your exercise program is very important!! It is also private and personal. Keep the odds in your favor. Think in terms of percentages. Know what a successful exercise program is. Remember, it's a program you can do week after week, month after month, year after year, and my favorite decade after decade, and never going over three weeks without getting to the gym! If something comes up and you miss it for a time, put it behind you and get back in there.

Number three is "I have no idea what to do." Well, I am going to lay out a proven method you can copy that should work for anyone. Gyms are all laid out in a similar way. In one section, you have "bikes and treadmills". Next, you have "Nautilus" type workstations, and finally, you have "free weights."

Number four is "not taking it seriously"! My hope is you will see or already know what is at stake in your success here! How much is it worth to be forty and feel like you are twenty-five? From the time you arrive till the time you leave; you are on the clock. Get your money's worth!! Don't spend your time visiting with people. If someone wants to talk, just continue to work and listen. Set your time limit and stick to it. As I have said, mine is thirty-five minutes. I will explore the time element later and its importance to your success. So, you will see the results you desire.

5

Key Number One Time

Remember the three critical key elements of a successful exercise program? Remember the definition of a successful exercise program? Now it is time to get into the meat and potatoes of it! Number one is "TIME". To me, this has many references. Time to get away from your busy life to get away to the gym. Time that you will put in year after year. And then simply the Time or length of your workout. These are crucial considerations that will increase or decrease your chances of success. Ask yourself are you going for a month or two or the decade after decade?

The first thing to do is select the days of the week you will exercise. Select the best time for you to get away from your life and the best time for you to be in a good state physically to get the best workout possible. Starting out, you should get three to four workouts a week. Select your days and stick to them. Everyone in your family should know your schedule. Your wife calls and says your brother-in-law is in town, and you must go to dinner. What do you say? But honey, it's Tuesday! And, of course, your wife will know you are at the gym every Tuesday at six pm. So, she will say, we will move it back an hour, and since your workouts are short and compact, this will work! What if your workouts lasted two hours? Are you seeing how important the time length of your workout is?

If your workouts are thirty-five minutes long, what are the percentages that you will have a successful exercise program? If your workouts last an hour, how far down do your chances go? How far down does it go if they last one hour and thirty minutes? Are you seeing the importance of Time here?

When you have your days to exercise selected, plan your entire week around those days; if you need to, mark your calendar. If you want, it will help to keep records. On the days of your workout, you should be rested. Plan your meals or snacks around your workout. As a person trying to be healthy, I always tried my best to eat healthy meals and snacks. Walking into that gym, you should be rested and ready to quickly get your money's worth! And use that time wisely! Push yourself! In a bit, I will show you how to grade your workouts. The goal is to walk into a gym and go away with a Grade 1 workout. Not sure what a Grade 1 workout is? Not just anyone can do it. But I can tell you it is an amazing feeling! Most people who regularly attend gyms will never experience a Grade 1 workout. But I will teach you how to someday walk into a gym and achieve it every time you go! This should be very motivating to you. This should put you in a place to be open to a program that will allow you to do what it takes to achieve success.

I can't talk about Time without discussing the subject of the use of "free weights" or Nautilus Stations. Keep in mind the goal we are working towards! Health! That is the goal! We are not going for muscle or lifting large amounts of weight. Although you can definitely get some muscle tone doing this. We are working on a program that will stand the test of time. Free weights have disadvantages when it relates to Time. There is no way I could do the exercises I do in thirty-five minutes using free weights. With the Nautilus Stations, I can rip through them with no trouble.

Another issue with free weights is in regard to the "start/stop" phenomenon that occur in the course of exercising. Using Nautilus Stations, you can skip a week and come back to the gym with ease. Using free weights, it's not always so easy. Soreness and injuries are common. The company I worked for offered a free membership to a local community center. A close friend told me he wanted to start going there to exercise. I tried to tell him how he should go about it. His reply was that he was old school and had to use free weights. I wanted to say to him that in two weeks, he wouldn't be attending the community center any longer, but he would find that out soon enough.

Let's say, for argument's sake, the percentage for success using Nautilus Stations is sixty-five percent, and using free weights is fifteen percent. I don't have actual figures to give you, but I do have thirty-five years of experience. Hey, I wish I was twenty years old and had the time to use free weights. I would be so hard you could roller-skate on me.

Here is some info on the subject. Both Nautilus machines and free weights have their own advantages and can be beneficial depending on your fitness goals. Here's a quick comparison:

Nautilus Machine

Safety: Machines provide a controlled range of motion which lessens the chance of injury.

They allow for concentrated isolation of targeted muscle.

Ease of use: Machines are easier to use and require less technique making them accessible to all fitness levels.

Cons:

- Limited range of motion.
- Less engagement of Stabilizer muscles.

Free Weights
Pros:

- Free weights mimic natural movements.
- They allow for a wide range of exercises and movement patterns.
- Free weights can be used for a variety of training styles.

Cons:

- Higher injury risk
- Free weights require more technique and knowledge to use effectively.

Which is Better?

Choosing between Nautilus machines and free weights depends on your goals and experience level. What is our goal? To have a successful exercise program that can be used decade after decade.

Now to get back to Time. For twenty-some years, the gym I attended was a thirty-minute drive away. I went there after work. My workout days were Tuesday and Thursday. I chose Tuesday so I would be rested from the weekend. Occasionally I would make the drive on the weekend to get a workout. But mostly all those years, I was getting two of these quick, short workouts and stayed in shape. This is a huge advantage.

How can this be, you might ask? I was in good health from all the prior years of having a somewhat healthy diet and exercising regularly.

6

Key Number Two Energy

Energy will define your success in your program. Without it, you will give up on your dreams of being healthy and accept whatever life throws at you. That is why so many systems fail. And that is why something like I am presenting will put the odds in your favor. This is why you choose to do the quick workouts and allow time to bring the things you want, such as muscle tone or weight loss.

Let me give you an example. About the time I got into my late fifties my employer changed our work hours from five eight-hour shifts to four ten-hour shifts. I had a thirty-minute drive there and back, so I basically had an eleven-hour workday. Then when I got off work, I would go to the gym and work out. At first, it wasn't so bad, but when I hit sixty, it started to be an issue because I would be tired from working long hours. Because of this, I had to force myself to go. Why go under these circumstances? Well, let me explain.

So, this brings us to another huge factor to help you have a successful exercise program all through life, even as you reach old age. It is called "The Stretch"! The first thing you do when you get to the gym is to get a good stretch in. It only takes three to four minutes to do. A good stretch session will get you primed to put in a good workout. So, my point is even though I would be tired from the long hours, all I had to do was get to the gym; once there, all I had to do was get a good stretch in, and then I was good to go for a good workout. Sometimes you just won't feel like exercising, but for me, most of the time, all I had to do was get there. Once there, "The Stretch" would put me in the mood or presence of mind to get a good workout.

As I mentioned earlier, I want to talk about forcing yourself to go to the gym. Normally, getting there is just a habit for me. I have done it forever and reap the benefits. Not doing it is just not an option. But for a few years, like I said, I had to force myself to go even though I was working long hours. Eventually I got to the age it just wasn't feasible. Luckily, about that time, a gym opened up in my hometown.

So, I was able to move my workout days from Tuesday and Thursday to Friday, Saturday, and Sunday. With these light workouts you can do them day after day with no problems. So, for me, the decision to miss a workout was if I felt like I couldn't get a Grade 1 workout, I wouldn't go in.

This reminds me of a situation I encountered years ago. I had a neighbor kid who did some work for me occasionally. I picked him up one day, and he mentioned he was watching TV all night. It was the summer, and he wasn't in school then. So, we worked about four hours doing landscaping-type work. I went to drop him off at his house, and he mentioned he would run a couple of miles and then work out. Now, being young can do great things for a person when it comes to energy, but you can take things too far. Lol! Your workouts should be far too important just to waste one. Sometimes you just have to wait till tomorrow. My point is when your workout day comes, be ready for it.

So, when it comes to energy, of course, diet is a key component. I always tried to eat healthy wholesome foods as most people do. But it can be tough these days. One thing you can always do is not overeat regarding portion size. I always think of it in terms of: In one hour from the time of eating, can I be at the gym and get a Grade 1 workout? And that's how I look at every meal. If I eat a medium-sized pizza alone, I won't be at the gym in one hour working out. So, this a good practice you can use.

One thing that is easier to control is your choices regarding snacks. I was always good at choosing healthy snacks between meals. Eat three lighter meals with good healthy snacks in between. Your place of employment can be the easiest place to do it because your choices are more limited there. Writing this makes me realize I could improve in this department now. We constantly have to keep ourselves accountable. Bringing into remembrance the habits that caused us to succeed.

My favorites were always baby carrots and sliced apples with peanut butter. Celery with peanut butter. Raw broccoli or cauliflower. Real food which is grown from the earth.

Some may want to eat something specific before a workout, like complex carbs such as whole grain cereals, whole wheat toast, or fruits. Drink plenty of water to stay hydrated. I never did anything special before a workout because I always thought of it as a full-time job to do these things. We are creatures of habit, and the earlier you develop good habits, the easier it will be to hold onto them. Like I said earlier, I would always plan my week around my workout days. Making sure when that day came, I was rested and had good energy because of my habits. When you are a really busy person, taking time out to get your workout in is of utmost importance. You should hold it in very high regard. You paid for your membership, so go get your money's worth! I need to mention that one thing I always tried to do after a workout was make a good protein drink. And this brings me to the next area of importance to a successful workout program. And that is the importance of good supplements.

I started taking supplements about the time gyms started popping up around the country. It was in the eighties, to early nineties, when there was a big push for everyone to get healthy. The movie "Perfect" comes to mind with John Travolta and Jamie Lee Curtis. I was in a small town in the Midwest, so it was nothing like that for me, but there was a definite push for people to get healthy as people could see the benefits of eating healthy and exercising. One thing that was so important to me was that, at an early age, I learned to listen to my body.

Your body is constantly feeding your brain with information; you can ignore that information or take note of it and use it to your advantage. I was always really good at that. Being able to recognize if a supplement is working or not. The issue with good supplements is they are very expensive. I can't imagine my life without them, now and in my past. Your health is a mix of a lot of things.

And all these different parts add up and are a part of the big picture. In my younger days, I had bad allergies, a lot of sore throats, and congestion. When I reached my mid-thirties, I put all these things together: the gym membership, eating healthy, and supplements, and I took care of those issues.

I was a person who always responded well to good supplements, more so than others. I have researched this and found that the body's ability to absorb and utilize nutrients can affect how well supplements work. Factors like age, gut health, and the presence of nutrients can influence absorption. I am sure you can apply this to over-the-counter and prescription drugs similarly. Overall lifestyle, including diet, exercise, sleep, and stress levels, can impact how well supplements work. Healthy habits can enhance the effectiveness of supplements. Genetic differences can affect how well individuals metabolize and respond to certain supplements.

Something I want to stress is the fact that when you pay for expensive supplements, you should see clear evidence that they are working. It goes back to listening to your body and knowing whether something is good for you.

Anyway, to summarize the subject of energy and its importance, just realize you need to have the best diet you can get, eat healthy snacks, and if you have access to good supplements, take them. And I want to stress doing this over a lifetime as opposed to doing it for a short time to get a healthy high. If you can put all these things together, it will pay off handsomely, I guarantee it!

7

Key Number Three a Good Plan

Now we get into the actual workout I use. To get the most out of these workouts, it is of the utmost importance for you to understand how I grade them. There are three possible grades. Grade 1, Grade 2, or Grade 3, with Grade 1 being the goal to reach. Grade 3 is taking your time and taking notes if you need to, which I definitely recommend. Noting the start time, following the list of stations, the sets, and the number of reps. You should do two sets at each station and try to get at least twelve to twenty reps on each set. At the end, note the time, and make some notes as to how it went. Mark the day with a grade. Completing the workout is a Grade 3. Don't be concerned with being seen walking around with a notepad or clipboard. I see it all the time. One thing I have always witnessed at every gym I have attended is they feel like a non-hostile place. People are busy doing their own thing and usually keep to themselves. No matter your circumstance or state of health feel good about yourself. You are doing a good thing. The other people you see there are doing the same thing. We are all a work in progress. It's not a competition!

To make a Grade 2, you must go through all the stations in around thirty-five to forty minutes and feel like it was a good session. After a few weeks or months, you should be able to make a Grade 2. If you are stuck in Grade 3's, consider taking out a station or simply continue as is. This is your program, so make it work! And keep at it. When your gym day comes around, be there. Learn to listen to your body. Do you need to go for more days? Do you need to come for fewer days? Remember, there are big prizes waiting for you when you make it work! If something comes up and you have to stop, no problem. As soon as you can get back in there.

Grade 1 workouts! WOW! This is what it is all about! The difference between a 1 and a 2 is how you feel at the end of the session. When you finish with the treadmill at the end and walk away, you should know beyond a shadow of a doubt that you just did something very good for your body. It is a great feeling and proves you are pretty healthy. If there is any doubt, it is still a Grade 2.

When you get a 1, you will know it. If you are stuck in 2's, it means you need to work on your breathing, intensity, energy levels, number of reps, and number of sessions a week. For a busy, normal adult, three to four of these sessions a week should be the max. But it all centers around your energy levels. Are you listening to your body? If you can do more than four fine. Your body will tell you. Are you learning how to make energy?

Remember, a Grade 1 requires a good amount of stamina, and it may take you some time to get there. And a 2 will get you some muscle tone and feeling healthy. What if it took two to three years of attendance to get there? Would it be worth it? Absolutely

How to do it: It starts with the stretch. The key to having a successful exercise program is being able to show up consistently for your sessions. If you don't do the stretch your percentages go way down! There will be days you don't feel like exercising, and you may want to stay home. However, in many cases, you can get to the gym, stretch, and then you are primed for a good workout. Remember, you are on the clock! It should last anywhere from two to four minutes. Think of it this way, a Grade 1 stretch will get you primed for a Grade 1 workout. If you can't do the stretch and you are stuck in Grade 2's, it might be something to reconsider.

Next, you are ready to move to your first station, the **Treadmill**. If I could only have one piece of equipment out of a gym, this would be it. As far as I know, no bike or stepper can compare to it. And you can do various positions on it to maximize the effort. It is vital that you push yourself here as it is for a short time! In the first minute, start with your feet at a wide stance, stepping forward with your stance about equal to your shoulders. Watch the timer and adjust the speed as needed, always holding onto the handles and pushing against them with your feet. There is a technique to this; if you want Grade 1's, you better find it. Minute two, move your feet in line with each other, one foot in front of the other, pushing against the handles. Minute three, move up close to the front and make fast, normal steps, side by side. You won't be able to push with your feet as much, but that is ok. If you feel like it, you can high-step it here.

In minute four, slow it down a few notches and continue with normal steps, still at a decent pace, cruising. In minute five, slow it way down to cool off and relax. At the end of five minutes, stop and move directly to the next station. Remember, you are on the clock. Do not excessively talk; this is serious business. Rest only if you have to between stations.

Next you are looking for the **Leg Extension** machine. Set the positions of the seat and weight you think will work for you and get two sets of around twenty to twenty-five reps. For this one, you really want numerous reps. After you do the first set, get the next station ready. Adjusting the seat or whatever it needs and weight selection. This speeds things up. When you are just starting out, you must find your own pace, always improving. When you are done with one station, the next one is ready to use. You can substitute one set of this with a Leg Curl machine. It is a good one also.

Next, look for a station called the **Shoulder Press**. These machines should be labeled at any reputable gym. If you can't find a particular station, ask the manager. Like always, two sets with at least twelve to twenty reps. Whatever feels good to you? There is a purpose to each of these stations. Learn technique. Get your money's worth!

Next up is the **Seated Bench Press**. Two sets, twelve to twenty reps.

Next up, **Lat Pull Down.** This one has a long handle; you can grip it wide or with your hands close together. This is one you want to try to get twenty reps and, of course, two sets like all the others. And, of course, always concentrating on your breathing. This whole workout is to focus on your lungs. A steady pace.

Next up **Reverse Curl Pull Down**: Or some type of curl. This will be on a tall stand with a cable hanging down. Just find an attachment you like, and this is one you definitely want to get at least twenty reps.

Now you are ready to go back to the **Treadmill** to finish out. For this set, you should use the same speed but at a **more aggressive pace** with your feet. It is vital that you understand this! The goal is for you to be **feeling really healthy** now. You just need to repeat the sequence you started with at a higher pace. And you are done! Congratulations! How you feel after you step off the Treadmill is how you grade your workout. If it is a Grade 1, you will know instantly! You will know beyond a shadow of a doubt that you just did something really good for your body! You will know that you are on the right track to achieving your goals regarding your health! It's based on your stamina. If it feels like a normal workout, there is something you need to work on.

Do the exact same workout year after year. I have been doing it forever. Going to the gym is just a natural part of life for me. I reap the benefits every day. As I said earlier, there were some years when I had to force myself to go after working a ten-hour day. That was when I was around sixty years old. But I still did it. The only way to do something like that is to know something about energy, fuel for the body, and how to use it.

You should always ask yourself what your health will be like in five years. What about ten years? Well, I know. I will be going to a gym somewhere and getting Grade 1 workouts.

8

Summary

Choose your time wisely! You can never get it back. Choose the food and snacks you consume with one thing in mind: energy! Become a technician at every aspect of your workout, from the stretch to each station you use at the gym. Evaluate where you are each day. Do I need to back off on intensity today, or am I at one hundred percent? Always listen to your body. It is talking; are you listening?

My hope is that you can appreciate what I have laid out here. It is a process you can follow from any level of health, progressing in laid-out steps. If you are not progressing, you should be able to examine what I have written here and find the solution to advance to the next level. Your number one goal is to strengthen your heart and lungs. Do this; with time, they will take you to your desired health!

The next work I hope to do is on Supreme Health for Life. Do you know what supreme health is? Can you imagine having it for a lifetime? I could talk all day about it, but I need to close it down for now. Thanks for reading, and best of luck with your exercise programs.

If I can assist, you can email supremehealthforlife@ya-hoo.com, and I will try to get back to you. You can also look for the website supremehealthforlife.

www.ingramcontent.com/pod-product-compliance
Lightning Source LLC
Chambersburg PA
CBHW051720250726

48653CB00008B/3122